The DIY SPUD FIT *Challenge*

A how-to guide to tackling food addiction with the humble spud.

ANDREW TAYLOR
& Mandy van Zanen

THE DIY SPUD FIT CHALLENGE

Website

www.spudfit.com

email

spudfit@gmail.com

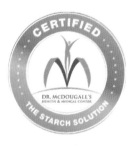

DISCLAIMER

I am not a doctor, nor do I claim to be any kind of health expert. The information contained in these pages is the result of my own research as a layperson, and of my direct personal experiences over the course of this year (2016). If you choose to follow the information here, you should do so *under the supervision of your doctor. This is especially important if you are on any medication* - it is quite common for health to improve so rapidly and dramatically on a whole foods plant based regime that continuing to take medications can become dangerous.

CONTENTS

FOREWORD

Andrew Taylor is the latest in a long line of people, spanning thousands of years, to discover the life-sustaining properties of the potato. This oft-maligned food is frequently equated to 'spoonfuls of sugar' or looked at only in terms of its carbohydrate content. Yet the potato is a powerhouse of nutrition. Some nutritionists have called potatoes a 'superfood'. Andrew calls them 'megafood'. The value of potatoes go far beyond the vitamins and minerals they possess. Potatoes contain all that is needed to sustain human life in pristine condition for months on end. But potatoes do not just help us to survive, they help us to thrive.

The world gasped when Andrew Taylor announced his plan to eat only potatoes for an entire year. "Surely he will quickly fall ill?!" His story spread around the globe as TV and radio stations picked up on his plan. Andrew's frequent YouTube videos quickly went viral as people everywhere tuned in to watch as the obese, depressed bloke with the Australian accent metamorphosed into a delightful, inspiring athlete.

Andrew's journey was not just about weight loss or eating potatoes. It was a journey of self-discovery. An attempt to reestablish his relationship with food. A self-described 'food addict', Andrew wanted to remove himself from the daily grind of choosing what he should eat and when he should stop. With a potato diet, one simply eats until full and eats again when hungry. It's impossible to overeat when potatoes comprise nearly 100% of your food.

Our modern world, full of tasty, addictive foods, has led to generations of people who simply do not know how to eat right. Snack-food manufacturers have us believing that artificially colored and flavored treats made of highly refined grains and oils are 'healthy'. This has led to a spate of eating disorders, obesity, and declining health in all who partake of this 'Westernized' diet. Andrew shows us how to use a simple, mono-food diet to reset our relationship with food, hunger, and the emotional responses to food.

Tim Steele, MSc,
Author, Amazon #1 Best Seller, *The Potato Hack: Weight Loss Simplified*

INTRODUCTION

I've been overweight my whole life. Even as an elite junior marathon kayaker I was always 5 - 10 kilograms overweight. It was probably the difference between me being one of the best paddlers in Australia and one of the best in the world, but no matter how hard I trained or how hard I tried to eat better, I was always overweight.

Over the years I've tried every diet imaginable and in particular I've tried really hard to get better at the idea of 'moderation'. I've tried eating less and moving more, I've tried the soup diet, paleo, juicing, green smoothies, low carb, eating for my blood type (and my personality type), calorie counting, points systems, weighing food, home delivered pre-packaged meals. I've even tried being hypnotised. Many times I've been successful for a few months at a time, lost a decent amount of weight and felt good about my achievement. But nothing has ever worked in the long term.

The time would always come when I'd be feeling good about the way I'd been eating, feeling like I had everything under control. Then sure enough there'd be some sort of occasion where there was cake, or pizza, or some other kind of junk. I'd tell myself "one slice won't hurt, just have a slice and get back on the diet tomorrow!". One slice probably wouldn't hurt - if it really could be just one slice! But of course it was never that way; sometimes I could eat one slice that night but then it would play on my mind for the next couple of days until I gave in and had two slices. Then a few days later I'd eat a whole pizza and then a day or two later I'd do it again. "Just one slice" was always the top of a very slippery slope back to my old destructive ways of eating. Soon enough I'd put all the weight back on plus a few kilos extra, and the feeling of helplessness would get that little bit stronger.

A moment of clarity

One afternoon in November last year I was sitting at home on the couch contemplating yet another failed attempt at weight loss. I was lamenting the fact that I have failed consistently at this throughout my life: why couldn't I just eat junk in moderation, like normal people?! Thinking about how my attempts at dieting always seemed to play out in the same way, I was suddenly struck by how similar this behaviour pattern was to that of an alcoholic or a drug addict. We've all heard stories of the alcoholic who goes for a few months without a beer and then one night says "I've got this under control now, just one beer won't hurt". But just one beer inevitably turns into a dozen or more until the alcoholic wakes up in a pool of vomit with no memory of what had happened to get them there. If my behaviour mirrored that of an alcoholic then it seemed reasonable that I had the same problem: I was a food addict! It hit me like a tonne of bricks. It was obvious - why hadn't I thought of this before?!

The healthy eating conversation always seems to start and finish with moderation. But what if some people aren't equipped for moderation? What if there is a significant portion of the population for whom moderation just does not work? Everyone seems to agree that the best course of action for an alcoholic is to quit drinking entirely and never do it again. Can you imagine someone recommending a heroin addict try moderation? Of course not - what a completely absurd idea! So why do we always seem to recommend eating junk food in moderation? I would bet my life that every single obese person in the world has tried to embrace moderation as a concept and has failed miserably at it. That's a lot of people.

If it's so obvious that a drug or alcohol addict would be best served by complete abstinence, I wondered: could I treat my food addiction the same way? Obviously we can't quit food entirely, it's unhealthy to stop eating. But I wondered if I could get as close as possible by quitting all foods except one. Was there a single food that could provide me with all the nutrition I needed to keep healthy and fit in both mind and body? I felt sure that if I could *remove the entire decision making process involved in eating*, I could give my mind a break from the constant internal debate that lead up to each and every meal. I felt sure that imposing an extremely boring diet on myself would force me to retrain my brain to get comfort, enjoyment and emotional support from other areas of life.

But why potatoes?!

The first thing to look at is their nutritional content. Contrary to popular belief, potatoes are extremely nutritious. Everyone knows they've got carbohydrates but they also have all the protein (6-8% of calories) and fats (2-3% of calories) we need to thrive. With a variety of different types of fibre and also a good amount of resistant starch, potatoes are excellent for gut health too. The humble spud also contains all the vitamins and minerals we need to keep us healthy and fit, we really can get everything we need from them! The key point is that we need to eat enough of them to get all the nutrition we need. As with any diet, if we restrict our intake and allow ourselves to go hungry then we won't be getting enough of one or more nutrients. If you listen to your body's hunger drives and eat until full whenever you feel hungry, then you'll do just fine eating potatoes.

Next we need to look at historical evidence. A number of foods could theoretically meet our nutritional needs in a similar way to potatoes but what's the story in reality? Throughout history potato-based diets have helped entire populations to thrive. The best example is the Irish diet of a few centuries ago. Up until the potato famine, the entire Irish population lived on a diet of almost entirely potatoes, almost all of their nutrition came from spuds and they thrived. Over the course of two centuries they maintained excellent health and their population boomed until the potato famine hit.
The Okinawan diet is also a good example to follow. Okinawa has the highest percentage of centenarians in the world. Their traditional diet is based on sweet potatoes, which provide well over 90% of their calories and they thrive on it, maintaining excellent health and vitality well into their eleventh decades!

There are also lots of examples of prisoners of war being fed only potatoes and maintaining excellent health and fitness for the duration of their incarceration, while also reporting feeling satiated by what they were eating.

My favourite example of this is an experiment from the 1920s, where a male and female marathon running couple were observed eating an all-potato diet for six months. They maintained excellent health and reported that they weren't sick of eating potatoes and in fact were quite happy with their diet. To top it off they ran personal best marathon times at the end of their experiment!

So it was settled, potatoes were my food of choice: and the SpudFit Challenge was born!

But a whole year?!

My original plan was to try eating only potatoes for a couple of months, but by the time I'd finished my research and made my decision, there were only a few days left until the new year. So like any good, experienced dieter who tells themselves "I'll start my diet on Monday", I decided to wait until January the 1st. Over those few days waiting to begin, the idea came to me that I could try doing it for the whole year!

I really can't explain where the idea came from. Eating only potatoes for a whole year was an extremely daunting thought, but for some reason I was drawn to it. I didn't know why I wanted to do it. To be honest I thought it was probably a bad idea, but I just couldn't shake it. I was sure that my physical health would be okay, but I thought that mentally I probably wouldn't be able to cope. But over those few days the idea gnawed away at me. I was really drawn to the notion of taking an entire year off from the burden of thinking about food all the time. I wondered about how different life would be if I could focus on things other than the psychological battle that was constantly raging over what I should eat for my next meal, for an entire year! I wondered if it was even possible. I thought I wouldn't be able to do it but I also thought that the only real failure in life is in not trying. So why not give it a try?

THE RULES

At the beginning of the year I decided on some rules to follow. I thought it was important to have a set of very simple, clear and easy to understand rules in order to bring this as close as possible to the experience of an alcoholic quitting the drink. An alcoholic has one rule: don't drink alcohol. Since I still had to eat food, my rules would be a little more complicated than that, but it was important to keep it as simple as possible. Every time I've reached that point in time where I thought "one piece of cake won't hurt", there was always an internal dialogue happening. We all know what it's like: the devil is sitting on one shoulder telling us to eat the cake, just this once, while an angel is on the other shoulder telling us that it's a bad idea. The devil has a whole heap of excuses and bargaining tools at his disposal, while the angel just knows it's a bad idea. Eventually the devil wins and we eat the cake and start the downward spiral.

I wanted to find a way to quiet the devil. If the rules were simple enough and clear enough then there'd be no cracks left anywhere for the devil to drive a wedge into my thoughts. The internal dialogue would go something like this:

(*Devil*) "Come on, just one piece of cake won't hurt, you can get back on your diet tomorrow!"
(*Angel*) "Cake is not potato, go away."
What other arguments could the devil then come up with? Conversation over.

RULE 1 - *Get medical supervision.*

This was my wife Mandy's rule actually - I originally had no plans to get medical supervision. When I first told her of my idea she was very supportive and trusted that I'd done the research and knew what I was doing. She knows me better than I know myself and she knew that this was not a decision I would have made lightly. Still, she wanted the peace of mind that comes with medical check-ups and blood testing by someone who really knows what they are doing. She fully supported what I wanted to do, but only if I gave her that.

Of course she was right as usual; any major change in diet and lifestyle should be supervised by a doctor - even if they totally disagree with what you're doing they can still check your vitals and do the blood work to make sure things are going well. I still believe that the most important measure of health is how you feel, but it's important with something like this to have the numbers to back you up, ***particularly if you're taking regular medication to manage a specific condition***. It is quite common for certain illnesses and medical conditions to improve so quickly when doing a Spud Fit Challenge, that continuing to take medication can become dangerous. ***This is vitally important for anyone on diabetes or blood pressure medications.*** Don't be surprised to see rapid improvements in these! ***Please*** take this seriously and be careful.

RULE 2 - Eat potatoes!

Initially I planned on eating only white potatoes for the entire year, but on meeting with my doctor I was convinced to include sweet potatoes too. This diet was not something that Dr Malcolm would prescribe to anyone, but he was very supportive nonetheless and happy to supervise me. Initially he suggested I add some greens to the diet but when I refused he suggested adding some sweet potato. I know that sweet potato is from a different family than white potatoes, but since it was still called potato I decided I could accept that! So the rule became to eat all kind of potatoes, including orange sweet potatoes and Japanese purple sweet potatoes.

To help feel less daunted by the idea of eating only potatoes for a whole year, I decided to allow myself some basic flavourings. I included herbs, spices and fat free sauces like tomato sauce (ketchup), BBQ sauce, chilli sauce etc. A little salt would be fine too, as well as a bit of oil-free, plant-based milk for making mashed potato. All of these things were to be kept to a minimum though; the purpose of the flavourings has been to keep things just interesting enough so as to not go totally insane from boredom.

The only nutrient that I had concerns about getting enough of from potatoes was vitamin B12, so I decided to supplement that with a mouth spray. Other than that I would take no supplements at all.

I think that more important than what I *can* eat, is what I *can't* eat. Strictly off limits are isolated oils such as olive oil and coconut oil. No fatty sauces such as mayonnaise, sour cream or aioli. No other pure fat foods such as butter or margarine, no cheese, milk or dairy of any kind and no 'low fat' or 'lite' versions of any of these either. No bacon bits or chicken or fish - absolutely no meat at all. Not even any high fat whole plant foods such as avocado or olives, nuts or seeds (or butter made from them). While the latter are healthy, for someone like me, they're high in fat and it's simply too easy to fall into the trap of eating too much.

What You Can Eat	What You Can't Eat
Potatoes	Oils, (including coconut and olive oils)
Sweet Potatoes	Dairy (no milk, cheese, cream or yoghurt)
Salt - minimal	Meat (including chicken and fish)
Pepper - minimal	Fatty plants foods like avocado, coconut, nuts, seeds and products of these foods.
Herbs - minimal	Anything that's not mentioned on the left!
Spices - minimal	
Fat free sauces - minimal	
Fat free dressings - minimal	
Low fat plant based milk like soy, rice or oat milk, just for making mash or adding to coffee	

RULE 3 - *Do not restrict or count calories!*

From all the research I had done it was clear that it is close to impossible to eat too many potatoes: the high level of fibre and water content in them means that they have a low ratio of calories to volume. If I simply ate as much as I felt like eating, whenever I felt like eating, then I was sure I'd get all the nutrition I needed and that my hunger signals would be switched off well before I ate too many calories. I resolved to never count calories other than for interest's sake. I would never weigh my food or count numbers of potatoes. I would not restrict my caloric intake in any way - and not just because I didn't need to in order to avoid gaining weight. Our worst eating decisions are usually made when we are hungry, so I reasoned that if I tried not to go hungry then I'd have fewer opportunities to make bad choices.

How to choose toppings

When thinking about toppings the first thing to remember is that this isn't about trying to make your potatoes delicious so you want to eat them all day every day. It's important to keep toppings very minimal, just to add a little bit of flavour to what you're eating. As a general rule, things like tomato sauce (ketchup), BBQ sauce, chilli sauce, sweet chilli sauce, sriracha, are okay. Vinegar and balsamic vinegar are okay too and many salad dressing are fine too. There are so many possible toppings and combinations of toppings that it's impossible to list them all here, so I'll give you some guidelines for choosing your own:

- Herbs, spices, salt and pepper are all fine.
- Sauces should contain no animal products at all. No milk solids or powders, no whey, no bacon bits, no cream, cheese, no egg, nothing that came from an animal.
- Sauces should contain no oils. No coconut oil, no olive oil, no oils of any kind whatsoever.
- No fatty plant foods at all. No avocados, nuts or seeds.

WHAT TO EXPECT

The Spud Fit Challenge experience will vary from person to person. A lot depends on what your diet was like in the lead up to beginning your Spud Fit Challenge. A lot also depends on what your personal health was like in the lead up. Of course the status of your emotional and psychological relationship with food will also play a big part in how you experience the Spud Fit Challenge. All of these factors will affect the intensity of the symptoms you experience, so just keep that in mind.

In the beginning you can expect some classic detox symptoms as your body adapts to an extremely clean diet. These could be things like a headache, nausea, sweating and body odour during days two and three. Bloating, gassiness and constipation could also be a factor around days four and five. Naturally these things are not fun to deal with but we need to see them as a welcome sign that our bodies are dealing successfully with something they aren't used to and so they are busy with working out how to handle the situation. Chances are your digestive system isn't used to the amount of fibre you are now taking in and is also not equipped with the appropriate intestinal flora to get the job done (your gut flora is a direct result of what you eat and is changeable as your diet changes - potatoes will give you excellent gut flora!).

My advice is to stick with it and listen to your body. If you're feeling nauseous and bloated, you probably don't feel like eating, so don't eat. Your body knows what's best so all you need to do is pay attention. Imagine the microbiota in your digestive system saying "Woah, what's going on here? Why didn't anyone tell us we're switching to a healthy, high fibre diet? We're totally unprepared! You're going to have to slow down while we get things in order down here!". So for a couple of days you might not eat much and you might not feel so good, the key is... don't stress! Just relax and eat as much as you feel like eating, also drink plenty of water. Over two or three days you can expect that your system will adjust, your hunger will gradually (or quickly) return and you'll be feeling better. You'll start eating more and your energy levels will increase. Your body is an incredible machine that can adjust to get the best out of any situation - you just need to get out of the way and allow it to do its thing. Don't second guess it, don't try too hard to figure things out, just sit back and listen. If your body says eat, eat. If your body says don't eat, give it the time it needs to get the job done. When you get through this initial period of adjustment, your body will start thanking you in all sorts of ways, like mine has.

Once you're through that initial adjustment period things will start to really happen for you. Again, results will vary between people according to your particular diet and health status in the lead up. Some things you can expect early on include better sleep, better mental clarity and weight loss.

If you go for longer than a couple of weeks you can expect to see improvements in your cholesterol readings, blood sugar levels and blood pressure, amongst other things. You may start noticing that some aches and pains in joints start going away as your body becomes less inflamed. Your energy levels will be boosted and your powers of concentration will improve along with your mental clarity. The boost in your serotonin production may also mean your mood improves over time. Best of all, you'll notice that your cravings for junk foods will dissipate over time, especially if you apply the techniques I explain later.

Heightened emotional sensitivity

At some point in the first few weeks you can expect to experience a state of heightened emotional sensitivity. As you move through the initial stages of your Spud Fit Challenge, you'll begin noticing how often you would normally reach for a snack without thinking about it. When you've had a hard day you'll realise that the desire for junk food is a coping mechanism. There'll be times when you find yourself thinking about or searching for junk food with no particular reason behind it other than habit. These times can be confronting because you suddenly understand just how much you've been relying on food to get you through the day. You'll understand how much you've been using food to push your emotions to the back of your mind, and since you have limited experience in processing strong emotions without the aid of junk food, you might have trouble dealing with these emotions. This might be the hardest part of all. But it's also the best part. This is where the real change comes from. Don't hide from the emotions. Face them, feel them, let them overcome you. Let the tears flow, try to experience these emotions fully. And then allow them to pass. Over time you'll get better and better at this and find yourself more comfortable and more at peace with yourself and your surroundings. You'll learn to deal more effectively with your emotions. You'll appreciate them as an experience that only adds to the richness of life.

BUT WHERE DO YOU GET YOUR...?!

I guess this is the time to answer the questions of people who are curious and/or worried about where various nutrients come from on the potato-only regime. The first thing to consider is the length of time you plan on doing your Spud Fit challenge; for anything up to a month there is very little chance you'll develop a deficiency that you don't already have - even if you eat nothing at all and drink only water! There are people who undertake water fasts for a month or more without being troubled by deficiencies, so we can be sure that eating potatoes is perfectly safe for that amount of time. But what if we want to go longer? How can that be healthy?

The number one question I get is, wait for it...

But where do you get your protein?!

I've got good news for you. There has never been a recorded case of protein deficiency in someone on a diet of natural foods, who was getting enough overall calories. *Never.* We seem to have an unhealthy obsession with protein and there doesn't appear to be any good reason for it. The World Health Organisation recommends we get at least 5% of our calories from protein. Around 6-8% of the calories in potatoes come from protein, which is more than enough to keep fit, healthy and strong (or even stronger!). The protein in potatoes is a complete protein too, providing a good amount of all the essential amino acids that are required by the human body. Basically, if you're eating enough total calories then you're getting more than enough protein.

But where do you get your iron?!

Potatoes have provided me with more than enough iron; if you're getting enough total calories from potatoes then you're getting way more iron than you need. I eat 3.5 - 4 kilograms (around 8 lbs) of potatoes a day and I'm currently getting over 500% of my daily recommended iron intake.

But where do you get fats?!

From potatoes! 2-3% of the calories in potatoes come from fats, and in a good balance of omegas. There is a lot of current research around that suggests that the ratio of omega 3/6/9 fats is more important than the total amount of fat, and potatoes have fats in the correct ratios. Importantly they also have no saturated fat at all - which is part of the reason they are excellent for lowering cholesterol.

But where do you get your calcium?!

From potatoes! There is quite a bit of calcium in potatoes but this is actually one area where potatoes don't quite meet the recommended daily intake. The strange thing about this is that all of my blood tests have shown my calcium levels to be on the high side. DEXA scans have also shown that my bone density has gone up slightly over the course of the year and remains well above avergae. A big reason for this is that when we remove animal products, oils and other processed junk foods from our diets, the body is able to function more efficiently and effectively. When we only take in clean fuel we get better at extracting everything we need from the foods we eat and we also get better at using every last bit of nutrition that's available, so that far less calcium than normal will be excreted in urine, resulting in perfectly fine levels of calcium.

But where do you get vitamin C?!

From potatoes! (see a pattern developing here?!). Potatoes are very rich in vitamin C - I'm currently getting more than 600% of my daily vitamin C requirements. This is another thing that simply isn't worth worrying about unless you aren't getting enough total calories - in other words, unless you're starving yourself, then you are getting enough vitamin C from spuds.

But where do you get fibre?!

Again, potatoes have provided me with more than enough fibre. Chances are that if you are eating only potatoes you are getting more fibre than you got from your previous diet. Potatoes also contain a nice diversity of fibre types, meaning they are excellent for gut health through promoting the growth of good microbiota.

There are many more questions to answer but I'm going to leave it up to you from here as I'm trying to keep this book short! If you're still worried then I suggest you use an online nutrient tracking app to see what's going on with you. In the past I've used Cronometer, and it has helped me to understand just how simple it is to get all the nutrients we need. You should also pay attention to your blood tests, but most important of all is to pay attention to how you feel. There is no better indication of health than how you feel. If you still feel like you need some extra individually tailored help, then contact me to book a personal coaching session.

HELPFUL HANDY HINTS

Communicating with friends and family

It's important that we do whatever we can to make this as easy as possible to complete. We need to do whatever we can to remove any barriers to success we might have. The first thing to do is talk to the people around you about why you are doing this. Explain your relationship with food and how it hurts you. Be open and honest with them and explain that you'd love their support. If you usually do the cooking then ask your partner/housemates/family to do their own cooking for the duration of your Spud Fit Challenge. Explain to them how much it would mean for you to not have to focus on preparing foods you can't eat.

Friends love to joke around and make fun of each other about all sorts of things - usually it's part of what makes friendships so great. Doing a Spud Fit Challenge is no different. Have this same open, honest discussion with your friends too. Once they know how strained your relationship with food is, how much pain it causes you, I'm sure they'll want to help you rather than make fun of you. If you go to a friend's house ask them to cook some potatoes for you - nothing could be easier than throwing some spuds in the oven! If they don't want to help then maybe it's time to rethink your friendship!

Communicating with your doctor

It's important to get your doctor to monitor your health, especially if you are on medication. It's very common to see dramatic health improvements very quickly, to the point where continuing to take certain medications can become dangerous. Ideally your doctor will be knowledgeable about nutrition and be supportive of a whole foods plant based diet, if not practise it themselves. Even better would be if they understand the amazing nutritional benefits of potatoes and are supportive of your Spud Fit Challenge. If your doctor doesn't fit the above description then it would be a good idea to try to find someone who does.

Of course I know this isn't always possible for everyone. If that's the case for you then you'll need to think about how best to communicate with them. Your doctor may advise you against the Spud Fit Challenge, which is totally understandable for someone who has been indoctrinated with mainstream, industry-funded education and marketing systems. In this situation there's no point getting angry or upset. As with your friends and family, try talking openly and honestly with them, explain how food affects your life and mind and tell them what you're hoping to get out of this. Ask them to Google me and see how well things have worked out for my health. If all else fails, calmly explain that you are going to try the Spud Fit Challenge anyway and that all that you want from them is to monitor your health. Ask them to think of it as an experiment.

Ask them to check your:

1) blood pressure
2) Fasted total cholesterol (including LDL and HDL)
3) Fasted blood sugar
4) Iron
5) U+Es (renal/kidney health)
6) Weight
7) LFTs (liver health)
8) Ca/MgPO4 (calcium, magnesium, phosphate)
9) Whatever else your doctor thinks is relevant and/or is worried about

Prior Preparation Prevents Piss Poor Performance

We make our worst decisions when we are hungry - not just food related decisions, but decisions in general. Our brains run on sugar, and when we are hungry we are also low on sugar, which means our brain is low on fuel and our decision-making ability is affected. On top of that, being hungry is a stressful thing - especially for someone who has a troubled relationship with food. It's uncomfortable to be hungry, which is good and perfectly natural - because that's exactly what drove our ancestors to search for food! So naturally we want to do whatever we can to change the situation. Of course, unlike our ancestors, we aren't in any danger of actually starving to death, but our subconscious doesn't know that, so a mild form of panic sets in. At this point in time we are likely to eat just about anything in an effort to make the hunger go away. Most people seem to think that we simply need to be tougher and stronger of mind and learn to fight off the hunger. I say that that's a losing battle; the best way to deal with that situation is to be prepared with healthy food - in this case, potatoes, ready to eat at all times. Cook big batches of potatoes at night and take them with you in containers everywhere you go during the following day. Remember: we are absolutely not restricting our caloric intake in any way, so if you're hungry, eat as much as you feel like eating! Always have potatoes with you. Always.

The right environment

It's human nature to want to stay within our comfort zone, waiting for the opportune moment to make the changes we need to make. We want transitions to be smooth and easy and for everything to go just perfectly the first time we try. Unfortunately, for most of us, the opportune moment never comes. Many people I've spoken with this year have talked about how their environment makes it very hard for them to stick to their healthy eating plans. I have absolutely no doubt that this is true. However I also have no doubt that for most of us it's close to impossible to change our environment.

We need to focus on the things we can control - and since we don't have ultimate control over our external environment, we need to work on creating the right environment in our minds. If we can learn to understand ourselves and our cravings, then we can gain control over our internal environment and therefore render the external obsolete. The following is aimed at creating the right circumstances for success in our minds:

Dealing with cravings

I really haven't had any troubles with cravings since the first week or two; I seem to be very much in control at the moment. Initially it was hard though, so I'll share a few strategies that helped me through the early stages.

1. *Potatoes first*

When I craved something delicious and mouth-watering that I used to enjoy, I would simply say to myself "you can eat whatever you like - after you eat a big plate of potatoes". That was an easy deal to make. I wasn't telling myself that I could never eat that stuff again, so that relieved the pressure - and I really meant what I was saying to myself. The trick though, is that after I'd eaten a big plate of potatoes there was nothing else that I actually wanted, so then it was easy to say no to the craving because it was gone! It's pretty common for people to say that you should never go shopping on an empty stomach because you'll end up buying a whole heap of stuff that you shouldn't eat. I'd like to extend that though and say that you should never even think about food on an empty stomach! Fill up on something healthy first - in this case potatoes - and then see what you crave.

2. *Thanks Hollywood!*

When I got a craving for something bad, I'd think of this dialogue from a scene in the film The Matrix:

(*Trinity*) Please Neo, you have to trust me.
(*Neo*) Why?
(*Trinity*) Because you have been down there Neo. You know that road, you know exactly where it ends. And I know that's not where you want to be.

This fits perfectly with cravings for bad foods. I know exactly what those foods taste like, how I'll feel after I eat them, and the path of self-destruction they'll lead me down - even if I only have them 'just this once'. Every time I have the opportunity to eat something bad, I compare it to this scene from The Matrix and ask myself if I really want to find out how good life can be - or if I want to head back down the same, sad old road.

3. *What are we really sacrificing?*

We often think of giving up all those delicious and amazing foods as a big sacrifice and wonder if it's all really worth it. I like the saying 'if you don't sacrifice for what you want, what you want becomes the sacrifice'. So I remind myself that, what I'm really faced with, is a choice between two sacrifices: either sacrifice the delicious foods or sacrifice my long term health, fitness and happiness. When I look at it that way, the choice is easy.

Once I got through the first week or two, the cravings went away. So it's good to be aware that it's possible to make it through and be rid of them altogether. At this point in time, I don't feel like my relationship with food is going to change before the end of the year, any more than it already has. I really feel like the job was done months ago. At this point I'm just completing the year because that's what I set out to do.

Change your measure of success

There's no doubt that what we weigh is an important indicator of our overall health - but it's out of our control. We can't weigh less just because we decide we want to. In fact our level of desire for weighing less doesn't matter in the slightest when we step on the scales! I'm not saying you should ignore what the scales say, just that you shouldn't make it your only measure of success.

We need to focus our energy and our efforts on the things we can control. **The thing we have the most control over is what we put in our mouths.** Here, with the Spud Fit Challenge we have a very simple plan that we *know* will work if we stick to it. There's no need to worry about what's happening on the scales; weight can fluctuate by a few kilograms each day through changes in water content and food moving through the digestive system.

Our behaviours are what's important. Our actions decide our weight loss or weight gain. So if you feel you need a measure of success to motivate you, it follows that you should judge your success by your behaviours and actions and let the scales take care of themselves; basically if you get to the end of the day/week/month (year!) having eaten nothing but potatoes (within the rules), then you've succeeded.

Get Support

When I started this year I was the only person doing anything like this that I knew of, so I've done it all alone. You can too! However many people enjoy and benefit from support and advice from people who've been there and done that. It can also help to share the experience with others - knowing that you're not alone in your struggle can be very helpful.

There are a number of ways I can offer you support:

• Sign up to my *newsletter* at www.spudfit.com

- Book in for a **one-on-one coaching** session with me (via Skype/phone) www.spudfit.com/coaching
- Join **The Spud Fit Challenge**, the ongoing online support group that began in September 2016, at www.spudfit.com/spudfitchallenge
- Join the conversation for posts, videos, discussions and live Q&A sessions with me and guest speakers on the Spud Fit **Facebook group** at www.facebook.com/spudfit
- Check out my **YouTube videos** at www.youtube.com/c/spudfit
- I'm also on **Twitter, Instagram** and **Snapchat** as Spud Fit.

ENGAGING WITH EMOTIONAL EATING

Your mouth is watering and excitement is building in anticipation of the upcoming foodgasm. The most incredible looking chocolate cake is in the display. You know it's bad for you but it just looks too delicious to ignore - your diet can start tomorrow... It's a familiar story and we've all experienced it, but are we being fair on ourselves?

It's natural for humans to want instant gratification. We are pleasure seekers by nature and we are constantly bombarded with the message that food is one of life's great pleasures - which of course it can be unless you're like me and that food pleasure comes at the expense of everything else. I think we do ourselves an injustice when choosing to eat the junk food instead of the healthy option. We focus on the immediate experience in front of us and neglect the overall experience. We chase short term highs that lead to long term lows. But how can we avoid this?

When we think about eating the chocolate cake, we focus on the immediate experience of eating it. We focus on the taste, the texture and the fireworks shooting off in our brains while eating this gastronomic delight. But when we choose the cake what are we really choosing? Of course we have to acknowledge that eating chocolate cake is an amazing experience in the moment, but in the interest of fairness we need to acknowledge the other emotional experiences that come with it - we need to bring forward all of the associated emotions and experience them in this moment, before we decide to eat the cake.

So think forward to ten minutes after you've finished the cake. If you're like me then by then you'll be feeling a combination of guilt and shame. An hour later you might be feeling depressed over yet another failed attempt at making healthy choices. Why can't I just say no? Why am I so weak?

The next day you'll be feeling a little sluggish after your body has worked hard overnight to digest crappy food while also not getting the nutrients it needs to make you feel your best. In six months, having continued this behaviour two or three times each week (or each day!), you'll be heavier and more sluggish, more depressed and sicker than you are today. If we can bring all of these feelings and emotions forward and experience them fully in the present moment, only then are we being fair to the overall experience of eating the cake.

Think about all the thoughts, feelings and emotions that go with eating the cake. Think about the shame, regret, sluggishness, depression, weight gain and bad health that go with eating the cake and really engage with it. Let these emotions sit in your soul for 30 seconds and really try to experience them fully.

Now switch your focus.

Look at the plate of steamed potatoes. The oral entertainment during eating isn't going to be as exciting, there might not be the same fireworks in your brain, it's fine to acknowledge that. But think forward ten minutes and you'll be feeling proud of the healthy choice you made - your self esteem has already received a little boost. An hour further forward and you're feeling lighter and more energetic because your body is easily digesting healthy food.

The next day you'll still be feeling good about your choice and you'll have a little spring in your step from the extra energy and vitality your healthy choice has given you. Six months down the track might see you ten kilograms lighter with a totally different outlook on life. Your habit of making good choices on a daily basis has helped you lose weight, get healthy and improve your mood and self esteem. Life is vastly better for you now!

In the interests of fairness, we need to bring all of these emotions forward too. We need to experience these emotions and feelings as fully as possible in this present moment. Let these emotions sit in your soul and really connect with them for 30 seconds, engage with it fully.

Once you've been through this exercise and taken no more than a minute to fully engage with the emotions involved in your choices, you might just find the choice no longer exists.

BUT WHAT HAPPENS NEXT?

When the Spud Fit Challenge is over I plan on following a whole food, plant-based diet, along the lines of that recommended by some of the world's leading experts in nutrition science. Drs John McDougall, Neal Barnard, Caldwell Esselstyn, Dean Ornish, Michael Greger, Michael Klaper and others have been recommending this way of eating for decades now, with clear evidence to back them up! A whole food, plant based diet involves eating whole or minimally processed grains, vegetables, fruits, nuts and seeds, as close as possible to their natural state. It means excluding all meat, dairy and egg products as well as highly processed foods like isolated oils and sugars - and no protein powders either. I believe - and the evidence suggests too - that this diet will be the perfect way for a recovering food addict to eat. The most addictive foods around always contain high levels of fat, sugar and salt: while this way of eating keeps those three things to a minimum, it simultaneously gives you the biggest 'bang for your nutritional buck'.

I also remain aware though, that my relationship with food is something that will need constant attention, in the same way that any recovering addict has to always remain vigilant about their particular vice. Like any good marriage, if I want it to stay strong, healthy and happy long after the honeymoon period is over, I need to pay attention to what makes the relationship special. I need to pay attention to what makes the relationship work. I currently have no desire at all to 'cheat' on this relationship; I do think it would survive and prosper well beyond a 'cheat meal' or a even a 'cheat day', but I just don't see the point in that. Currently there is no desire in me to have even a tiny taste of chocolate cake or a doughnut. The food I've eaten this year has loved me back in more ways than I could ever have imagined, and my life is immeasurably better for the steadiness, security and deep love in this new relationship. The cheap thrills and momentary highs involved in dietary 'cheating' seem pointless. I am very much enjoying this new feeling about food, and I plan to continue nurturing this new relationship "til death do us part"!

FREQUENTLY ASKED QUESTIONS

Can I really eat as much as I like?

Yes! Not only can you eat as much as you like, you *should!* Our worst food decisions are made when we are hungriest so it's very important to avoid hunger. Potatoes are very high in fibre and water content, both of which contain no calories. This means they fill you up while keeping calories low. They also rate very highly in terms of satiety - they keep you feeling full for a long time. Don't overthink things; our bodies have evolved over millions of years to be very good at telling us when we need food. If you give it a bit of time your body will adjust to this way of eating and your hunger levels will adjust accordingly. Your body will make you just hungry enough so that you eat just the right amount to get everything you need.

What if I'm not sure if I'm feeling hungry or bored?

Eat! Again, try not to overthink things. Your only job is to eat potatoes when you feel like it and stop when you feel like stopping - that's really all there is to it! It doesn't matter if you're feeling hungry or bored or anything else; if you feel like eating then eat as much as you feel like eating and don't stop until you feel like stopping! Forget about trying to read signs and signals from your body, just eat when you feel like eating. If you eat when you're not actually hungry it just means you'll either eat less at your next meal or you'll wait longer until you eat again. Gradually you'll adjust and start feeling more confident about what you're doing and your body will thank you for it.

How much exercise should I do?

It's up to you. It's important to focus on the biggest problems first and for most of us food is the biggest problem! Changing the way you eat will have a far bigger impact on your health and fitness than changing the way you exercise. Focus on one thing at a time and make it the most important thing you do, the thing that will make the biggest difference in your life. Once you've settled in to the Spud Fit Challenge and are feeling comfortable with it, you'll probably find your energy levels have increased and you want to start exercising, that's the perfect time to start exercising! The best exercise plan is the one you can stick to so find something you enjoy. Go walking with an audiobook to help pass the time, that's something I love to do. As for how much, just do as much as you feel like doing, if it's a chore then it's harder to stick to.

Do I have to eat only organic potatoes?

Organic potatoes are better but if eating organic is a barrier to your success then don't worry about it. Personally I eat both organic and conventionally grown potatoes. You'll be far better off eating conventionally grown potatoes than you will a fast food meal or a plate of donuts! It's really important that we make this challenge as easy as possible to complete so if it's easy for you to get organic potatoes and it's within your budget then go for it. If not then relax and eat some conventionally grown potatoes in the knowledge that they are still extremely healthy and you're still doing great things for your body and your relationship with food! The benefits of eating conventional potatoes far outweigh the negatives of not eating potatoes at all! Do the best you can with what you've got.

How much water should I drink?

As much as you feel like drinking. Your body is amazing, it has developed an ability to tell you when to drink so you just need to learn to listen to it again. Just like eating potatoes, you should drink as much as you feel like, whenever you feel like drinking. You should also check the colour of your urine, you're aiming for it to be close to clear so if it's yellow then the first thing you should do is drink some water!

If it's yellow or straw
drink some more!
If it's clear or white
then you're alright!

What else can I drink?

Coffee or tea is fine as long as you don't use dairy milk, try a low fat plant based milk such as soy, rice, almond or oat milk.

Alcohol is obviously not a healthy choice but I'll leave that one up to you. For me food was by far the biggest problem in my life so I chose to put all of my focus and energy towards that, I worried that quitting alcohol at the same time as I quit food might just make the whole thing too hard so I decided to allow myself the occasional drink. Perhaps I'll quit drinking next year when my Spud Fit Challenge is over. I'll leave that decision up to you too, just be aware that drinking alcohol is not a healthy choice. No cocktails though, nothing mixed with juice, milk, cream or soft drink!

Apart from that you shouldn't drink anything else. No soft drink, juices, smoothies, coconut water or milkshakes.

How do you cook without oil?

Water frying works well depending on what you are cooking - put a small amount of water in the fry pan and fry like normal. Obviously it's easy to make boiled or steamed potatoes without oil. Baking is the same, just put them in the oven without oil. Use non-stick cooking gear. I love my granite fry pan (brand is Baccarat), it's really great for non-stick frying, even pancakes just slide right off. Waffle irons and sandwich (panini) presses are easy to find with non-stick coatings too.

What about going out?

When going out for dinner check the menu online to see if there's anything at the restaurant that contains potatoes. There usually is so then you just need to give them a call and ask them to prepare a big plate of steamed, boiled or baked potatoes. This is really easy and cheap for a restaurant to do so most of the time they'll be more than happy to help you out, it's easy money for them.

If you're going to someone else's house then ask them to cook some spuds for you, nothing could be easier for them than throwing some spuds in the oven for an hour. Alternatively offer to bring your own. You can still have a great time eating with friends and your Spud Fit Challenge will probably generate some interesting conversation.

Do I need to buy all the kitchen equipment?

No. You can do this just fine with a pot of boiling water. An oven is a bonus and so is everything else.

What should I have for breakfast/lunch/dinner?

Lots of people seem to struggle with the idea of what to actually eat for each meal, especially breakfast - it doesn't matter. Potatoes are edible at all times of the day and night! If you have to have something traditionally considered breakfasty (yes, I have the authority to make up words) then try potato waffles and potato pancakes from the recipe section of this book. Otherwise I say just make big batches of mashed, boiled or baked spuds at night and eat them throughout the next day.Do I have to eat the skins?

That's up to you. There's plenty of nutrition in potatoes, with or without the skins. I leave the skin on mine but mostly because I can't be bothered with peeling so many potatoes every day!

Do I need to supplement with anything?

Assuming you have no existing vitamin or mineral deficiencies then there is no need to supplement with anything to be healthy for a month of spuds. Many people are deficient in B12 though, regardless of diet, so it's worth checking that out. If you plan on doing this for longer than a few months then it's a good idea to get a B12 supplement, it doesn't matter which one.

Is it okay to use a microwave?

Yes. Use a microwave to heat your leftover potatoes or reheat them in a pot on the stove, whatever works for you. If you're hungry and you don't have the ability to heat your spuds, eat them cold. Cold potatoes aren't as good as hot ones but as my friend Tim Steele says in his book The Potato Hack - "If you aren't hungry enough to eat a cold, boiled potato, you aren't hungry!".

Can I use fresh herbs and spices, onion and garlic?

Yes... BUT... I prefer to use the dried and powdered forms. A big part of the Spud Fit Challenge is taking the focus off food as much as possible. That means reducing preparation and clean up times too and it means reducing the amount of time and brain space we have to put towards the food we eat. Throwing some dried onion powder in will literally take two seconds, while chopping, sautéing and cleaning up after preparing an onion for use takes considerably longer and a lot more thought.

How long do potatoes keep in the fridge?

I've always eaten mine within two days and they've always been fine. I cook big batches at night and eat them over the following day or two. I don't know how long until they go off though as I haven't actually reached that point.

What if I fall off the wagon?

Get back on! We all make mistakes from time to time, what defines us is how we recover from them. Mistakes are things that happened in the past. Leave them there. Don't waste any time or energy thinking about what you ate yesterday, or even an hour ago. What you eat next is all that's important.

FOREWORD TO THE RECIPES

I've enjoyed eating food over the course of my life. I've enjoyed it too much in fact, to the point that it became a problem. The point of my Spud Fit Challenge is not to try to find all the best, most delicious, interesting and amazing ways to enjoy potatoes within the rules I've set. The point is to 'quit' food - to take time off from using it as a crutch, for emotional support, comfort and enjoyment. I'm not obsessing over which recipe I'm going to try next, which combinations of herbs, spices and sauces I'm going to use or which cooking method. I've intentionally made my food boring so that I have to find ways to get emotional support, comfort and enjoyment from other areas of life.

I really do eat very simply - 95% of my meals are either mashed, boiled or baked potatoes with minimal use of some kind of flavouring that I decide on the spur of the moment. Often I just use a bit of salt and am done with it. For me this is not about being creative in the kitchen, it's about putting some good quality fuel in my tank and moving on with my life without using any more brain space on food than is necessary.

Having said that, I know a lot of people are approaching this from a different perspective and for some people the preparation of food for yourself or for others is a hobby outside of any food eating addiction you may have. For that reason I've enlisted the help of my beautiful and far more culinarily talented wife Mandy. This section belongs to her! She's going to take you through a few recipes that are still very simple and fit within the Spud Fit rules but are at least slightly more interesting than anything I have to offer!

Over to you Mandy...

NOTES ON THE RECIPES

Hi Spuddies!

Whether or not a 'recipe' section should form part of this book was a decision Andrew has to and fro'd on for quite a while; as he has already made very clear, the whole point of the potato-only diet (and the whole reason he arrived at the idea in the first place) was first and foremost to attempt to rid himself of a food obsession - it was a way to stop thinking about food altogether. In that way a recipe section seemed a bit counter-intuitive; although the recipes are exceedingly simple (they're 'created' by me after all!), they are slightly more complex, and therefore more time and thought-consuming, than simply boiling a pot of spuds and eating them. However there are a few factors that seemed to favour including them rather than leaving them out:

You don't have to use them!

These recipes, while slightly more fancy than Andrew's usual meals, are all Spud-Fit approved - there is nothing in these meals that isn't allowed on the diet Andrew created for himself, and you will see the same physical results as long as you stick to them. However as far as food psychology goes, simplicity really seems to be a key on this diet and if you struggle as Andrew always has with food choices, then you may benefit from keeping your meals as plain as possible - the advantages of this are obviously enormous.

You're not obsessed with food

If your problem is more that you've unknowingly been eating unhealthy foods rather than actually suffering from the effects of an unhealthy psychological relationship with food, it won't be a problem for you to try some more varied ideas and you might enjoy it enough to maintain a potato-centric diet in the long-term.

If you're getting bored

Many people have reported losing interest in food entirely on a potato-only diet (me included). But everyone is different and if you find yourself getting bored and tempted to stray from spuds only, perhaps trying something slightly more interesting could keep you on the path.

You don't exist in a vacuum

Many or most of you probably have jobs, families and friends with whom you share time. And some of that time is probably spent eating. Often your time and efforts might be spent feeding other people as well as feeding yourself. There are meals in this section that may come in handy in these situations - I can't think of many dinner guests turning their noses up at fresh gnocchi or kids refusing a big plate of waffles or chips for dinner!

People kept asking for recipes!

I can't tell you the amount of times Andrew has been surprised by an email or message asking him for recipes - he mostly just boils or bakes a big plate full of spuds and whacks on some sauce (yes it's as ceremonious to watch as it sounds!) so to him the idea of following a recipe was a puzzling one. But one day after another email came and he looked particularly flummoxed, I said "If people want recipes, why don't you just give them some?". So here we are!

SOME NOTES ON THE RECIPES

This is not a 'real' cookbook!

Andrew is very sweet about ~~everything~~ my culinary prowess but he really is deluded! That said, I am very much into fresh plant-based flavours, and all this really is is potatoes with fresh plant-based flavours. You kind of can't go wrong. There is nothing complicated here and absolutely nothing I am an authority on - they're just suggestions to give you some ideas and they're based on what I personally like. I won't be offended if you change them!

Forbidden 'fruit'

There are sauces included here where I have used foods (vegetables) that are not allowed on the Spud Fit Challenge. For example I have made a mushroom gravy for chips. There are two justifications for this (both Andrew-approved of course):

1. The sauces Andrew buys (chilli, tomato and barbecue mostly), are of course made from real ingredients (chillies, tomatoes and...barbecues?) in the first place - but through the cooking process they end up very concentrated and he uses them very sparingly. The exact same principal applies here: you are using real ingredients to make very concentrated sauces, and you should use them only sparingly - they're just to add a tiny bit of flavour.

2. What exactly was I supposed to do with a potato-only recipe book if I wasn't going to make my own sauces? Tell you to cook some spuds and then go to the shop to buy them in a bottle?! To be honest Andrew would have been (actually, is) okay with this, but it was just a little too fraudulent for my liking, so I told him that if he wanted me to do a recipe section I had to be able to make the sauces myself.

It's personal

All flavourings are to taste: I haven't included quantities most of the time. When I have they are based on my personal preferences. It's impossible to tell you how much you need to flavour your potatoes because a) I don't know how much flavour you like and b) I don't know how many potatoes you're using; the quantity needed to get full will vary wildly among different people (and who here has ever found recipe serving sizes to be accurate anyway?!). Also if you're attempting a full Spud Fit Challenge (potatoes only for a while) you may be cooking enormous batches ahead of time. Just experiment!
Don't like it? Don't eat it!

Leave out anything you don't like, obviously! If you can't do chilli, onion or garlic, please just don't use it! Interestingly, onion and garlic, while they will always be problematic for some, might be less so on a spuds-only diet once your guts have had a rest. Take it nice and slow though!

No, it's not bacon.

All of the recipes in this section feature Desiree potatoes. That's the box of spuds we had lying around the week I did the recipes and it's their pink skins that you're seeing in the pics - it's not bacon.

Anyone for fibre? You don't have to, but you may as well leave all the skins on (except for the gnocchi). There is lots of good stuff in the skins, especially fibre. Fibre is your friend (though if you're coming from a S.A.D. - Standard Australian/American Diet - you may take a little time to, um...get acquainted, if you know what I mean?). And as Andrew mentioned, peeling 3-4kg (8lbs) of potatoes a day would get boring pretty quickly! A very important note though: do not eat green potato skins. It can be toxic especially in big doses. Peel those ones.

WHAT YOU MIGHT NEED

For some of these recipes I've used a food processor, but you could easily make do with a decent knife and a cheese grater instead. You'll need a blender for some of them, but a cheapie will do if you chop the spuds or other ingredients pretty small first.

You will definitely need a non-stick pan as this is the only way to avoid oil when you're not water frying. Same with the waffle maker, though these are usually non-stick anyway. You have to season both of these items as per manufacturer's instructions otherwise you will probably come to grief (we've had to throw out an almost brand new waffle maker this year). I heated them up very high, spread a tiny bit of oil around and then wiped it off completely with a paper towel. This seemed to do the trick and the oil in your food is then virtually non-existent. Don't cheat, wipe it all off.

You will definitely need some kind of pot for boiling, a masher for mashing, and an oven for baking. I'm assuming you have a chopping board lying around, you'll need that.

SOME FINAL TIPS

- I've used fresh herbs in all of these recipes - apart from the fact that I just like them, a recipe book of just potatoes using just dried herbs would have looked a bit bland! I also used fresh garlic, ginger and lemon juice, but I used store-bought ground spices. Dried and powdered forms of any of these are perfectly great for cooking and are recommended when you're trying to keep your food as simple as possible.

- I've used commercial powdered veggie stock whenever stock is mentioned - look for no oil, salt-reduced, whole foods only where possible. If you want to make your own stock you can, but for me it was a step too complex given the points I've discussed earlier (simplicity is key).
- Always add salt (or salty sauces) last, right before serving so that it hits your tongue first.
- I have mentioned 'sautéing' a few times: I mean in water only, not in the traditional butter or oil.
- I've mentioned plant milk one or two times: try to find one that has no added oil - they usually add oil to plant milk to make them as fatty as even low fat dairy milk (i.e. this is the last thing you want).
- I've used flour a couple of times: Andrew was very strict on me using potato flour only (white or sweet). I've only found it in a handful of shops but you can find it online too (iHerb.com is a good resource).

Well that's more than enough from me! Let us know how you go, and Spud Up!

Mandy

RECIPES

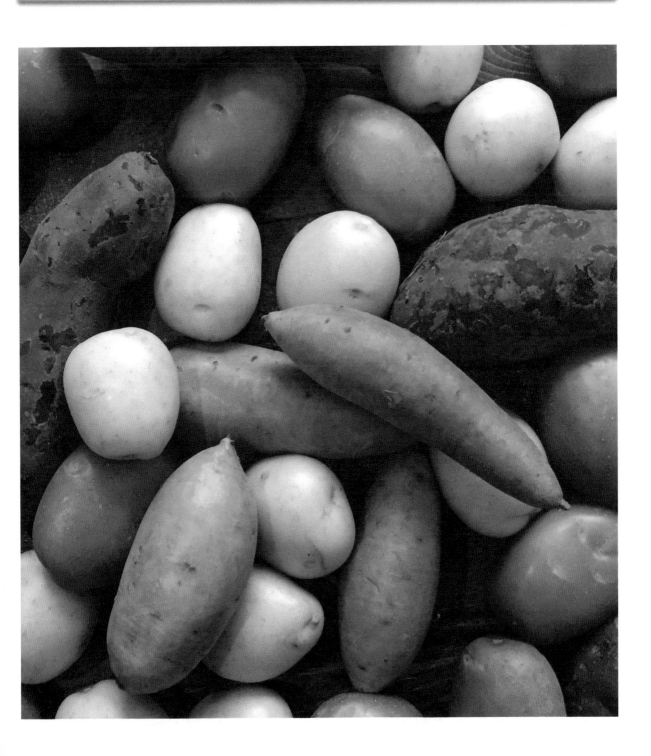

BOILED LEMONY SPUDS WITH CHIVES

(Almost) as simple as it gets!

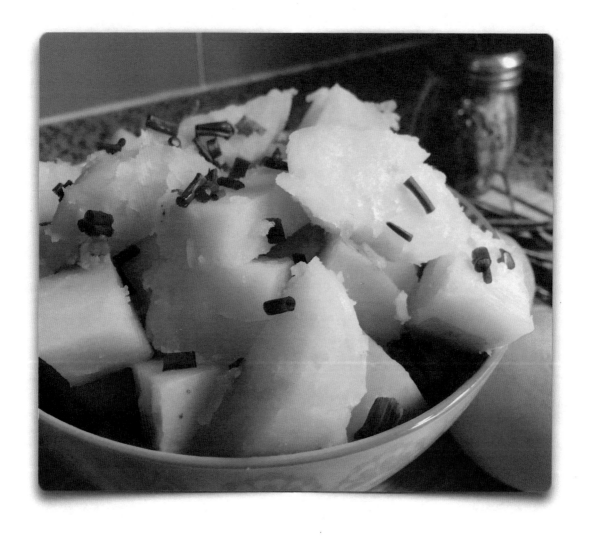

WHAT DO I NEED?

Spuds

Lemon

Chives

HOW DO I MAKE 'EM?

1. Boil lots of spuds - enough to fill your face and have plenty leftover for a few more meals.

2. Chop them into whatever shape you prefer.

3. Chop up some chives (or fresh herb of your choice if you're intent on defying the regime!) and sprinkle them liberally over the top.

4. Squeeze plenty of fresh lemon juice over the top of all of it.

5. Season to taste (we love this smoked garlic salt we found in a little market one Sunday, in the Blue Mountains, near Sydney www.smokeandspice.com.au).

6. Gobble them up!

BAKED HASSELBACK POTATOES WITH GARLIC, PARSLEY AND OREGANO

Guilt-free garlicky pleasure!

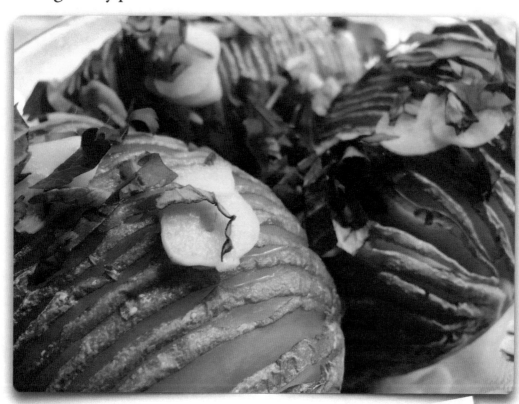

WHAT DO I NEED?

Spuds

Garlic

Parsley

Oregano

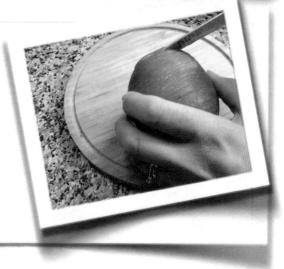

HOW DO I MAKE 'EM?

1. Slice a big pile of potatoes as thinly as you can from the top *almost* to the bottom, being careful not to cut all the way through.

2. Bake for 40-45 minutes on 180°C/356°F

3. Slice or mince some fresh garlic and sauté **in water only** with some veggie stock (don't add oil or butter or anything like that!).

4. Sauté long enough to soften the garlic but so there is enough garlic flavoured water left to pour over your spuds.

5. Finely chop some fresh parsley and oregano.

6. Take the cooked spuds out of the oven, sprinkle the fresh herbs over the top and then pour over the stock and garlic juice.

7. Season to taste.

NOTE: Baked spuds store well for a few days in the fridge but will lose their crispiness.

SPUD FIT'S SIGNATURE MASH WITH FINE FRENCH HERBS

Andrew's go-to favourite, but a bit fancy!

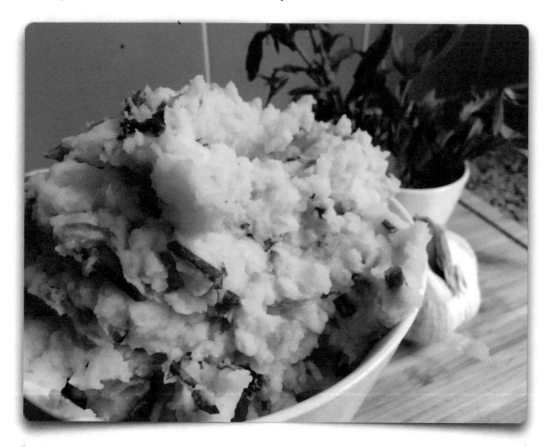

WHAT DO I NEED?	Garlic	Chives
Spuds	Plant-based milk	Parsley
Veggie stock	Nutritional yeast (optional)	Tarragon
Onion		Chervil

HOW DO I MAKE IT?

1. Boil lots of spuds until they are really soft (leave the skins on).

2. Mash them up as roughly or finely as you like.

3. Add stock powder, onion and garlic powder (or the real thing, sautéed in water first), and some nutritional yeast if you have it/like it.

4. Add a bit of plant-based milk (a light version, with no added oil) to make it easier to mash.

Now you have made *Spud Fit's Signature Mash*!

5. I add a finely chopped selection of fresh herbs (I *love* tarragon, chervil, parsley and chives) and stir through right before serving.

6. Season to taste.

So hungry writing these recipes.

NOTE: Mash will keep in the fridge for a few days and is okay for freezing.

GIANT CREOLE SPICED MASH CAKE

Just like mash, but better!

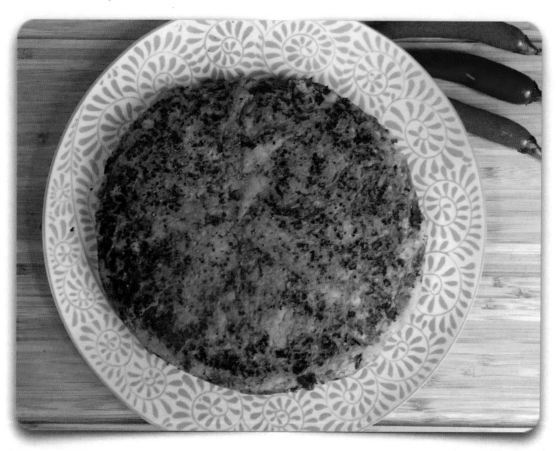

WHAT DO I NEED?	Onion (powdered)	Thyme
Spuds	Black pepper	Basil
Plant-based milk	Paprika	(Optional) Chilli - fresh or dried
Garlic (powdered or fresh)	Cayenne pepper	(Optional) Fresh lemon juice
	Oregano	

HOW DO I MAKE IT?

1. Boil heaps of potatoes.

2. Add enough plant-based milk (no added oil) to make mashing easy, but not so much that it becomes sloppy. It needs to be bound but pretty dry for this recipe to work. Mash away!

3. Mix in the other ingredients.

4. Heap a pile of mash in a non-stick pan (if necessary, coat it in a little oil and wipe it *all* off with paper towel before adding the potato).

5. Flatten across the pan into a big thick pancake.

6. Cook on medium to high heat.

7. After 4 or 5 minutes, check the underside.

8. When it's browned, put a large dinner plate over the whole mash cake, flip the pan upside-down so the mash cake falls onto the plate and then then carefully slide it back into the pan to brown the other side. It's important that it's browned enough on the first side before you flip it otherwise it will come apart. If it does, eat it anyway, it doesn't taste any different!

9. Squeeze lemon juice over the top.

10. Season to taste right before serving.

Yum!

NOTE: This will keep in the fridge for a few days but you'll need to recook it in a pan if you want the original texture. Better to just keep the mash and make a new mash cake.

CLEAR POTATO SOUP WITH CORIANDER AND CHILLI

Inspired by my obsession with Vietnamese phô, this clear soup just feels so healthy and satisfying. I often eat it for breakfast!

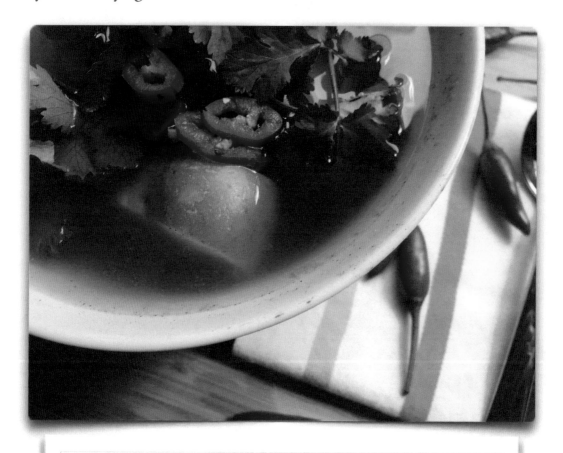

WHAT DO I NEED?	Onion	Chilli sauce (No oil! No fish paste!)
Spuds (there's a pattern emerging)	Garlic	Fresh lemon juice
Veggie stock	Coriander	
	Chilli	

HOW DO I MAKE IT?

1. Dig out the biggest soup bowl you own. It's probably not big enough for this, so go and buy a bigger one or use a bucket.

2. Fill it with water. Tip this water into a saucepan and heat on the highest setting. It will reduce during cooking and end up around about the right amount for the bowl when the potatoes are in there too (this recipe isn't much good for cooking ahead so just make it as you want it).

3. Add veggie stock.

4. Add fresh or powdered garlic and onion.

5. Cut up as many potatoes as you want to eat straight away (I eat two to three medium size ones usually) in whatever size and shape you find appealing. Put them in the water.

6. Bring to the boil and cook until the potatoes are soft enough to eat. Don't overcook as they'll flake off all through the broth and it won't have the same appeal. Not that that's the point of this whole thing anyway I suppose.

7. Pour the lot into your enormous bowl. At this point I add heaps of hot chilli (sriracha, yum!) sauce, chopped fresh chillies too, fresh coriander and squeeze lemon juice over the top.

8. Rise and shine! (with your glowing red chilli face, ha ha!)

NOTE: Make it fresh right before serving, though if you have pre-boiled spuds at hand this is a super-quick meal!

POTATO DAHL

If you don't have a food processor, you can finely chop your spuds by hand, or else just add the spices to a mash. Yum!

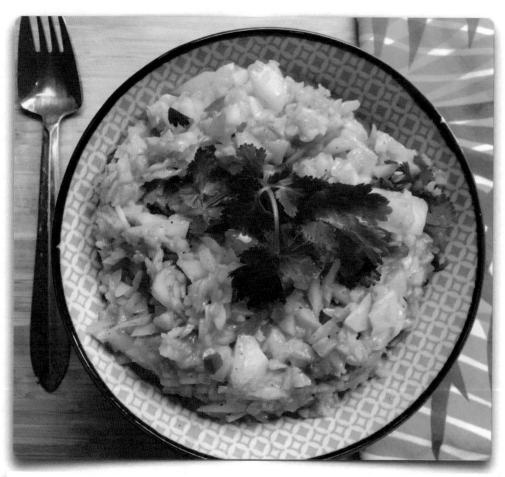

WHAT DO I NEED?	Ginger	Garam Masala
Spuds	Turmeric	(Optional) Fresh chillies, coriander and lemon juice
Garlic	Coriander	
Onion	Cumin	

HOW DO I MAKE IT?

1. You can make heaps of this ahead of time so start with a big pile of spuds.

2. Put them through a food processor to chop them fairly small, no smaller than grains of rice, but not too big either. If you don't have a food processor, chop pretty finely instead (or else just make a mash with the same ingredients).

3. Chop or mince fresh garlic, onion and ginger.

4. Cover the bottom of a big pan with water, bring to the boil and sauté them all together.

5. Add the rest of the ground spices. (Alternatively you can use an Indian spice mix).

6. As soon as they have all dissolved into the water, add the potato.

7. Add chopped red chillies if you like.

8. Cook until the potato is soft (the length of time will depend upon how small you have chopped the potatoes) and the water has been absorbed/evaporated (if you still have a lot of water but the potatoes are really soft, tip the excess water off).

9. Serve garnished with fresh coriander. And you may as well add lemon juice too because that stuff is ace.

NOTE: This can store in the fridge for a few days or be frozen.

POTATO RÖSTIS WITH SALT AND PEPPER

Delicious crispy morsels made without oil?! Shut the front door!

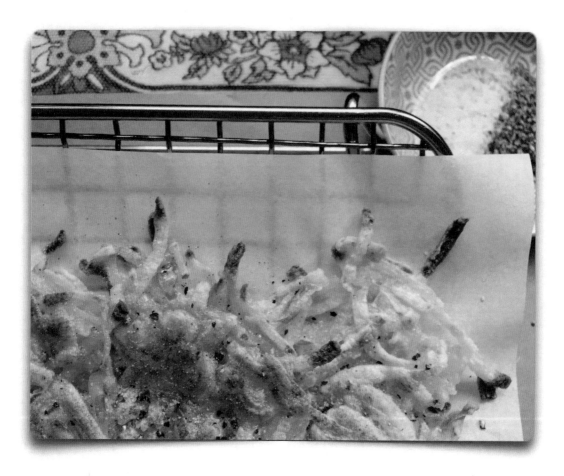

WHAT DO I NEED?   Veggie stock

Spuds

    Salt and pepper

Potato flour

HOW DO I MAKE 'EM?

1. Grate lots of potato (manual grater or food processor) and put it in a mixing bowl.

2. Add potato flour little by little, mixing with your hands.

3. Add water and flour alternately in small amounts until all of the potato is coated in the flour/water batter.

4. Heat a non-stick pan on high heat (you may need to season first, as per instructions at the beginning of this section).

5. Add small clumps of the grated potatoes in batter and flatten with a spatula. The thinner they are the better they will cook and the crispier they'll get.

6. When they're browned on one side, turn them over and do it again.

7. Serve hot from the pan with salt and pepper.

NOTE: The raw mix will keep for a few days in an airtight container in the fridge BUT the potatoes will oxidise and go grey. They're still fine to eat but a bit ugly.

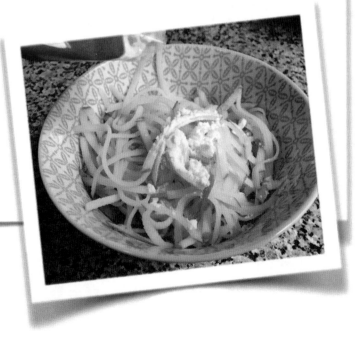

CHIPS WITH MUSHROOM GRAVY

Any Brits here? This is for you!

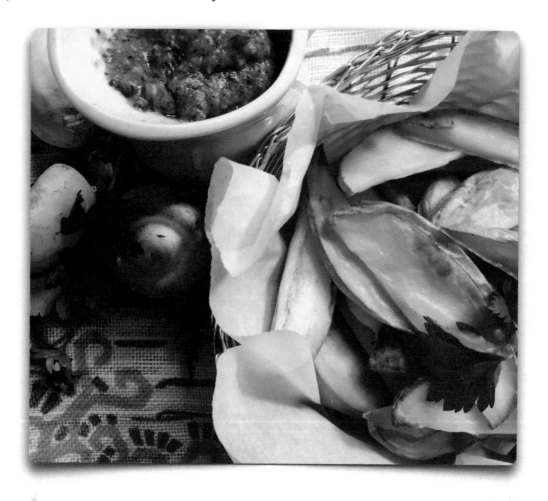

WHAT DO I NEED?	Onion	Potato flour
Spuds	Garlic	Parsley
Mushrooms	Veggie stock	Pepper

HOW DO I MAKE 'EM?

1. Preheat the oven to 180°C/356°F

2. Slice potatoes into wedges and arrange them in a single layer on a baking tray covered with baking paper.

The gravy:

3. Cover the bottom of a big pan with water and bring it to the boil.

4. Add veggie stock, onion and garlic (freshly chopped/minced or powdered) and mushrooms and sauté in water until mushrooms start to soften.

5. Add some sifted potato flour, little by little, waiting in between. It will eventually start to thicken and when it does it will happen quickly. You may need to alternate adding water and flour until it's the right balance of thick and runny.

6. Put the contents of the pan, the parsley and the pepper into a blender and mix on high. If it's very thick add more water - you want the final product to be a concentrated sauce full of flavour that is thin enough to flavour your chips but still able to be used sparingly.

NOTE: You can make a big batch of the sauce and freeze, or it will keep in the fridge in an airtight container for a few days.

POTATO WAFFLES WITH THREE RED SAUCES

Waffles: they make me think of The States (well after Belgium!).
This is for you!

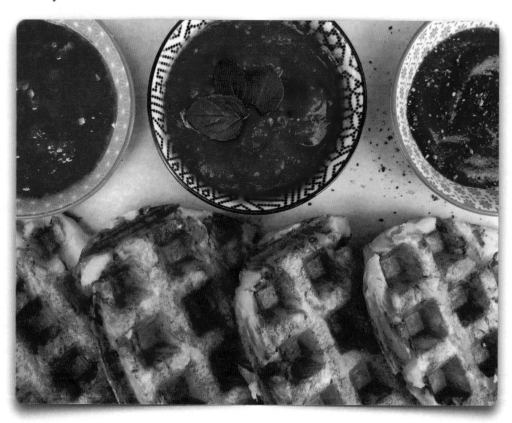

WHAT DO I NEED? Spuds! Chillies (about 150g/ 5 oz) Tomatoes (0.5kg/17 oz)	Tomato paste (plain, 2 tbs or just under 1 oz) Garlic Onion Vinegar	Pure maple syrup All spice (ground) Paprika Mustard (I used Dijon) Black Pepper

HOW DO I MAKE 'EM?

I have to be straight up with you - you need a waffle maker for this recipe. If you have that, these are easy.

Waffles:

1. Boil spuds until they are pretty soft but not falling apart.

2. Cut them in half lengthways.

3. Heat up a waffle maker as high as it goes. You might need to season it before each batch - see notes at the start of the recipe section.

4. Stick in one half spud per waffle square and squash the whole lot as flatly and as evenly as possible. You'll need to keep squashing further (perhaps with the aid of a tea towel) for much of the cooking process.

5. Leave for ages - at least 15 - 20 minutes I reckon (depends on your machine!). When you are checking, do so very carefully, as it's pretty much a case of no second chances with the fickle thing that is potato waffles. You need to be able to open the lid without them pulling apart. You can try some gentle hinting with a wooden implement or similar.

The sauces

Sweet chilli:

1. Place the chillies (half de-seeded), a clove of garlic and 1/2 cup of vinegar in a food processor (or else chop very, very finely).

2. Move to a saucepan or pan, add 1/2 cup of maple syrup. Bring to the boil then reduce to simmer until it has thickened.

Tomato sauce (ketchup):

1. In a saucepan combine tomatoes, tomato paste, garlic and onion and bring to the boil.

2. Simmer on low for quite a while (maybe half an hour?), stirring occasionally, until the tomato is very soft and has broken down.

3. Add 1/2 cup/4 oz of vinegar and 1/4 cup/2 oz of maple syrup, and ground All Spice to taste. Cook for another 20 - 30 minutes until it has all reduced and become 'saucy'. Blend if necessary.

Barbecue:

1. Combine some of your tomato sauce (above) with some mustard, sweet paprika and black pepper. Add more vinegar and maple syrup to achieve your desired taste.

TWO INGREDIENT GNOCCHI WITH NAPOLI SAUCE

This is really happening: you can be a Spuddy and still feed your guests something 'normal'.

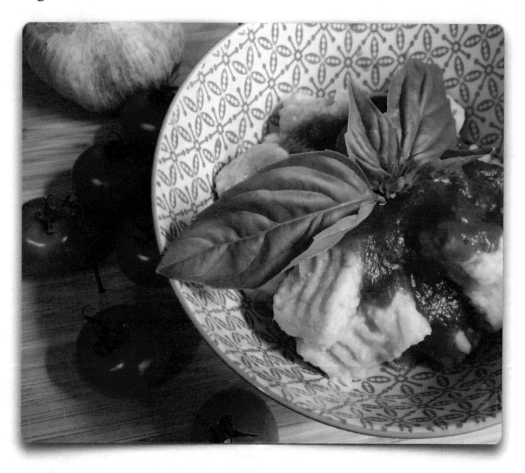

WHAT DO I NEED?	Potato flour	Garlic
	Tomatoes	Basil
Potatoes		

HOW DO I MAKE IT?

I'm glad you asked.

Gnocchi:

1. Boil and mash potatoes as per your (or Andrew's) favourite recipe. I like to add extra pepper for this, but that's a taste thing.

2. On a chopping board put a layer of sifted potato flour. It's not always easy to come by locally, so look for it online if you need to. I used sweet potato flour I had lying around for this recipe, so my gnocchi went a bit yellow.

3. Dump the mashed spuds on top and add a bunch more flour - start with a little and take it from there.

4. Knead the flour into the spuds with your hands.

5. Keep adding flour and kneading until dough begins to form - it took me a lot more than I anticipated.

6. Knead into a big potatoey doughy blob.

7. You may need to play around with quantities of flour and add some water until you get the big doughy blob.

8. Chop the blob into smaller blobs, roll those into sausages (or 'snags', as we Aussies say) and then chop the snags into small bits...like gnocchi.

9. If you're aesthetically-oriented you can push a fork into each one to make the stripes.

10. Boil a huge pot of water.

11. Drop the gnocchi in and make sure they don't stick to the bottom.

12. As soon as the gnocchi have floated to the top they are ready. Scoop them out and drain on paper towel.

Sauce: *in the meantime!*

1. Roast some tomatoes and fresh garlic cloves in a baking pan (no oil - use aluminium foil or baking paper) for about 15 minutes on at 180°C/356°F.

2. Remove from oven and put them straight into a blender with some fresh basil. OMG yum.

NOTE: Gnocchi can be made in advance and frozen.

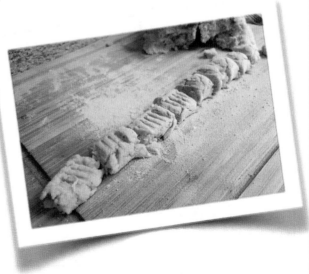

POTATO PANCAKES. YES, IT'S TRUE!

Buckwheat? Pfft. Just look at these beauties!

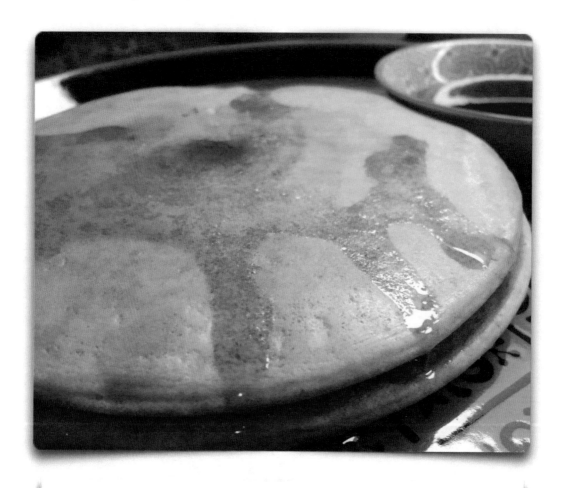

WHAT DO I NEED?	Maple syrup, cinnamon,
Spuds	nutmeg, whole food jam
	(jelly) or lemon juice to top.
Potato flour	

HOW DO I MAKE 'EM?!

1. Chuck some raw spuds in a blender and blend them to liquid. You may need to chop them up a bit first.

2. Mix in some potato flour and blend again until you've achieved a batter consistency.

3. Heat a non-stick pan or hotplate (high setting) and pour on the batter. You can cook them much as you would a pancake except that they take quite a lot longer to brown (as you're cooking potatoes).

4. Flip the pancake and brown the other side.

5. Top with pure maple syrup (no imitations) or lemon, cinnamon or nutmeg, whole food jam (jelly) - or your choice of Spud Fit approved topping!

NOTE: Pancake mixture doesn't store too well as it goes bitter, so it's best to make up only as much as you need.

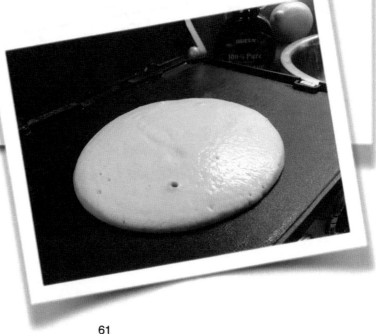

SWEET POTATO CHOCOLATE MOUSSE

No. Way. *Yes. Way!*

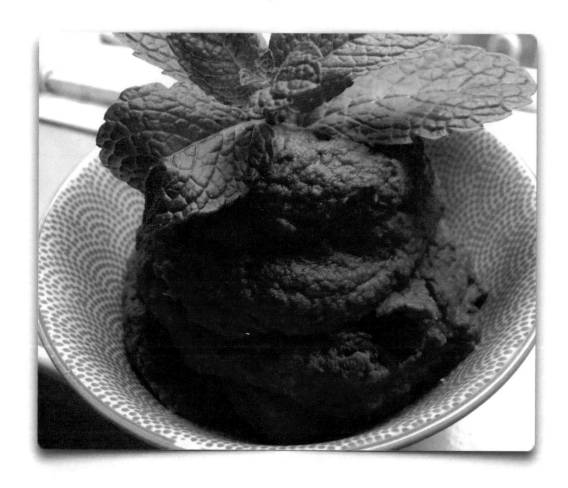

WHAT DO I NEED?

Sweet potatoes

Maple syrup (pure, not maple flavoured sugar!)

Pure vanilla essence

Cacao (or alternatively nutmeg or cinnamon)

HOW DO I MAKE IT? TELL ME NOW!

1. Peel and boil a few sweet potatoes.

2. Combine the maple syrup and a few drops of vanilla essence in a blender and whizz until smooth.

3. At this point taste it: it's so lovely and sweet - you might be content adding some nutmeg or cinnamon and be done with it, or else add a couple of spoons of cacao.

4. Blend and adjust ingredients to taste.

5. Pop in fridge to chill, serve garnished with mint.

Don't talk to me, I'm eating.

RECOMMENDED

SUPPORT

Sign up to my *newsletter*, book an *individual coaching session* and join *Spudtember* at www.spudfit.com.

Join the conversation for *posts, videos and live Q&A sessions* with me and guest speakers on *Facebook* www.facebook.com/spudfit

Check out my *videos* on YouTube www.youtube.com/c/spudfit. You can also find me on *Twitter, Instagram and Snapchat*.

STUDIES

Stanislaw Kazimierz Kon and Aniela Klein *XXXV. The Value of Whole Potato in Human Nutrition.* From the State School of Hygiene, Warsaw, Poland. (Received December 29th, 1927.)

Foster-Powell K. *International tables of glycemic index.* Am J Clin Nutr. 1995 Oct; 62(4):871S-890S.

Holt S. *A satiety index of common foods.* Eur J Clin Nutr. 1995 Sep;49(9):675-90.

Kofranyi E. *The minimum protein requirement of humans.* Tested with mixtures of whole eggs plus potato and maize plus beans. Z. Physiol Chem 351 1485-1493, 1970.

Caldwell B. Esselstyn Jr *Updating a 12-year experience with arrest and reversal therapy for coronary heart disease (an overdue requiem for palliative cardiology)*

Barnard, N. D., Cohen, J., Jenkins, D. J. A., Turner-McGrievy, G., Gloede, L., Green, A., & Ferdowsian, H. (2009). *A low-fat vegan diet and a conventional diabetes diet in the treatment of type 2 diabetes: a randomized, controlled, 74-wk clinical trial.* American Journal of Clinical Nutrition, 89(5), S1588-S1596.

David, L.A. et al. (2014). *Diet rapidly and reproducibly alters the human gut microbiome.* Nature, 505(7484), 559-63.

BOOKS

The Starch Solution Dr John McDougall

Prevent and Reverse Heart Disease Dr Caldwell Esselstyn

Proteinaholic Dr Garth Davis

The Pleasure Trap Dr Doug Lisle and Dr Alan Goldhammer

The China Study Dr T. Colin Campbell

The Campbell Plan Dr Thomas Campbell

The Low Carb Fraud Dr T. Colin Campbell

Whole Dr T. Colin Campbell

Dr McDougall's Digestive Tune Up Dr John McDougall

Dr Neal Barnard's Program For Reversing Diabetes Dr Neal D. Barnard, MD.

The Potato Hack: Weight Loss Simplified Tim Steele

DOCUMENTARIES

Forks over Knives

Plant Pure Nation

Food Choices

WEBSITES

Dr John McDougall's website https://www.drmcdougall.com

Dr Malcolm Mackay (my doctor) and **Jenny Cameron's** website http://www.wholefoodsplantbasedhealth.com.au/

Physician's Committee For Responsible Medicine http://www.pcrm.org

T. Colin Campbell Centre For Nutrition Studies http://nutritionstudies.org

Dr Michael Greger's videos on the latest in nutrition research http://www.nutritionfacts.org

The Potato Hack https://potatohack.wordpress.com/2016/03/13/potato-hacking-for-weight-loss-or-maintenance/

YOUTUBE VIDEOS

Here's the very first thing I saw when I first started researching the whole crazy idea of quitting food:

Potatoes: The perfect food John McDougall MD

A great video (that I'm featured in) to put your minds at ease on getting enough nutrients: **Nutrients Don't Matter - Don't Worry About Them**

The great Neal Barnard talks about diabetes: **Diabetes with a bold new dietary approach: Neal Barnard at TEDxFremont**

Why no oil? Let Dr Caldwell Esselstyn Explain: **No Oil -- Not Even Olive Oil! Caldwell Esselstyn MD**

Let Jeff Novick explain fats to you: **TO NUTS: The Truth About Fats (Jeff Novick DVD)**

Don't fear carbs!: **Sugar Don't Make You Fat - Fat Does! Dr. McDougall**